ESSENTIAL OILS

Essential Oil Recipes and Aromatherapy for Weight Loss, Physical and Mental Health

By Gerard Johnson

TABLE OF CONTENTS

Chapter 4 - Best Ways to Use Essential Oils

Vapor

Chapter 5 - How to Take Care of Your Essential Oils

Storage

Disposal

Reusing Old Essential Oil Bottles

Conclusion

Legal & Disclaimer

Legal & Disclaimer

The information contained in this book is not designed to replace or take the place of any form of medicine or professional medical advice. The information in this book has been provided for educational and entertainment purposes only.

The information contained in this book has been compiled from sources deemed reliable, and it is accurate to the best of the Author's knowledge; however, the Author cannot guarantee its accuracy and validity and cannot be held liable for any errors or omissions. Changes are periodically made to this book. You must consult your doctor or get

Introduction

Since time immemorial, essential oils and aromatherapy have been widely used in a variety of ways to achieve optimum health and wellness. From pain relief, meditation and even as part of beauty regimens, people have found them indispensible.

The use of essential oil dates back centuries ago. The earliest accounts experts were able to find dates back 18,000 BC. The evidences were discovered in caves somewhere in France. They were paintings depicting the use of herbs and oils as part of healing rituals.

Egypt, China and India were some of the other cultures that showed early use of essential oils. Much of the accounts gathered in the said countries depicted how valuable the oils are in today's practice of medicine.

Aside from health, essential oils became popular for spiritual healing. Egypt's priests, during their era, were the only people allowed to use oils in their covenant with their Gods. The Knights in Europe used the oil to ward off bad spirits.

Through time, more and more uses of essential oils and aromatherapy are being explored. Most of them have already taken the spotlight and have reached common knowledge. However, as the oils benefits can be limitless, this book aims to show you more about the oils than what you probably already know.

There are special considerations you have to make before buying any essential oil bottle you can get your hands on. Aside from cost, you also need to consider how it's packed, when it's distilled and tons of other factors. Taking a deeper research and understanding about these factors can help you land your hands to only the highest quality oils on the market.

Chapter 1

Aromatherapy and Essential Oil Therapy: The Differences You Need to Know

Aromatherapy is different from essential oils. However, this doesn't mean the two aren't interrelated. As a matter of fact, they complement each other- almost interchangeable actually.

Aromatherapy uses blends of essential oils, either by direct application, massage or inhalation, to elicit a response. In theory, aromatherapy can help in both body and mind healing. From mental relaxation and clarity to energy boosting, tons of people are turning to this approach in healing.

It actually isn't new. The use of aromatherapy and essential oils dates back to earlier civilization and culture. However, as the effects of these techniques are extensive, a lot of people have their interest piqued.

Essential oils, or quintessential oils, are extracts of plants often achieved by distillation. The most common method of extraction you'll find is the use of steam. Parts of specific plants are placed inside a device which is then placed above heated water. Lavender and peppermint oil are the most common ones extracted through this method.

Other means of extracting essential oils include expression and supercritical CO_2 extraction. Expression does not involve heat. Instead, it relies on mechanical means, such as grating, in extracting oil from a plant. CO_2 extraction, on the other hand, uses CO_2 to extract oil. The process may be similar with that of using distilled water. However, since CO_2 possess a different chemical property than water, the oil extracted may contain different properties and effects, too.

Aromatherapy relies on the use of essential oils. Because of this, they are often used interchangeably. The most common aromatherapy method you'll find is massage. The use of humidifier, compress and steam are also fairly common. Depending on your goal, there's a different aromatherapy and essential oil for you.

Chapter 2

How to Find the Right Essential Oils

Choosing the right essential oil is super easy. The key is to know your purpose. If you're feeling pained, find an essential oil that can target your aching muscles. If you feel stressed out, then you should look for an essential oil that has a calming and soothing effect. If you feel cramped and bloated, there's an essential oil that can help with your indigestion.

Doesn't sound complicated right?

The tricky part, however, is knowing what an essential oil can really do and how you should use it. An essential oil is not just about picking a bottle and lathering its content over your target area. It also isn't about using an oil and expecting an overnight miracle or a 'snap-of-a-finger' kind of effect. You have to know the best oil and the right way to use it.

To get the most out of aromatherapy and essential oil, you need to be thorough in doing your research. There are tons of oils that can basically do the same thing. Lavender and chamomile, for example, have both soothing effects but smell a tad different from each other. By reading and doing your research, you'll be able to narrow down the list to only the essential oils you need and want.

After knowing your preferences, there are other things you need to consider in picking the right essential oil. It includes:

- **Cost**

    In general, high quality essential oils can be costly. The price may be due to the tedious processing, packaging and distribution companies have to go through in order to keep the freshness of their products. However, you should note that not all expensive essential oils are the best. The cost may be a reflection of how concentrated or well extracted the oils are but if the marketing sounds too good to be true, be more critical.

- **Ingredients**

As much as possible, always make it a point to read ingredient labels. If you read something that sounds synthetic, don't buy it. To get the most out of an essential oil, it's best if you stick with the organic ones. "Unsprayed" is also a good term to find in products because it means that no chemicals have been splashed and sprayed over the plant sources.

- **Purity**

The purer the oil the more benefits you can get. However, as processing is necessary to keep the essential oils longer, most companies tend to process them to the point that the quality becomes altered. If you're going to buy an essential oil, make sure to buy from a trusted seller or from people who specialize in the craft. Buying directly from them means you'll be getting a valid product.

- **Label**

Aside from ingredient, scanning labels for distillation and expiry dates is also a must. You want to buy a product that's not only fresh but one that you can use as long as possible. It wouldn't give you your money's worth if you get a product that's going to expire in a few days, right?

Brand is also something you need to consider. When buying an essential oil, it can give you more peace of mind when you buy a product that's from a trusted source. Aside from brand, make sure to scan the label for the source, chemo type and the country it was distilled.

- **Packaging**

Packaging is an important criterion you need to consider when buying your bottle of essential oil. Bottles that are amber in color and those in blue are good choices. You should also steer away from buying essential oils that come with a rubber dropper in its container. Rubber tends to dissolve in the long run and can affect your oil's potency.

Instead of rubber dropper, try to find bottles that are secured with an orifice reducer. If you worry about how you can get a good amount of the product without a dropper, your next best option is to use a glass pipette. It's equally accurate without the risk of altering your essential oil.

These criteria are not only crucial in determining the quality of the essential oil. It can also give you an assurance that the product you're going to use on your body is safe and effective. Because there are a lot of misleading products in the market, you have to be extra cautious in choosing to avoid falling victims to scam and fraud. For added peace of mind, you can do a bit of background check to see if the seller you are dealing with sells legit essential oils. Aside from the seller, be sure to run a search about the brand and other consumers' review about the product. By knowing what other people think, you can get a good idea of what you should expect.

Chapter 3

Best Essential Oil Recipes for Your Different Needs

The best thing about essential oil is the fact that there's always one that can specifically meet your needs. In case you're still in the shadow about picking the right essential oil, here's a list to help you get a clearer idea of your choices:

Essential oils for losing weight

Essential oils are also helpful for people who want to lose weight. Although they can't directly take the extra inches off of your waist, they can still help you drop a few pounds.

Peppermint Essential Oil

Peppermint oil can help improve your digestion. It can help you feel full for a longer period of time. It also works to tame your appetite so you crave and eat less.

Peppermint essential oil has a direct effect on your serotonin production. It's the hormone that makes you crave for chocolates and other sweets. The lesser you eat these types of food means the lesser chance of putting more weight.

To use peppermint oil for weight loss, you can diffuse a few drops of the oil before meal time. You can also drop a small amount of peppermint in your bath for the same effect. You can also take peppermint internally by adding drops of it on a glass of water. Generally speaking, 1 to 2 drops is enough for one drinking.

Grapefruit Essential Oil

Grapefruit oil can prevent bloating by working against water retention. Aside from suppressing your appetite, it also helps break down body fats faster so it can be readily used for energy. It also has antioxidant properties to assist in flushing toxins, which can contribute to weight gain, from your body.

There are two ways you can use grapefruit oil for weight loss. The first method involves massaging the oil directly to a target area. It can be your arms, your thighs or your waist. To start off, you need to mix a few drops of grapefruit oil and a separate carrier oil. The most recommended for this purpose is olive oil. You need to massage the combined oil for around 30 minutes on the area and avoid washing it off after to achieve the best effects.

You can also take grapefruit oil internally. Before taking this step, make sure to buy an essential oil that's food grade. Add one or two drops of the oil in a glass of water and drink it preferably in the morning.

Lemon Essential Oil

Lemon oil essential is highly effective as an appetite suppressant. It works similarly with grapefruit oil in that its scent can help curb appetite. Aside from digestive health improvement, this oil is also helpful if you want to detoxify and flush off toxin build up in your intestinal track.

Because its scent can prevent you from fully indulging in your meal, you can diffuse its scent in your dining room. For an internal approach, you can add it to your water to detoxify your system. If you're plagued with cellulites, rubbing the oil on your problem areas can help lessen those stubborn fat deposits.

Bergamot Essential Oil

Bergamot has an indirect effect to weight loss. Instead of curbing appetite, this oil manages emotional cravings. Because stress is one of the main reasons why most people eat too much when they aren't really hungry, suppressing it can help avoid the excess weight. Bergamot is also rich in polyphenols. It can help you burn fats faster and easier.

If you're feeling stressed out, just grab your bottle of bergamot oil. Pour a few drops of it on a piece of cloth and take a sniff. The vapors should be able to calm you and your stress down. Aside from inhaling its scent, you can also rub the oil on your neck and your feet for an instant mood buster.

Essential Oils for Mental Health

Essential oils are highly popular because of their effect on human mental health. It isn't surprising as one of the earliest uses of these oils is in relaxation and meditation. However, as years went by, experts were able to establish a strong effect of these oils against stress, anxiety and even depression.

If you are experiencing any of these issues, then this list can help you improve not only your mood but your mental clarity and focus as well.

Lavender Essential Oil

Lavender oil has a soothing and calming effect by slowing down rapid brain wave activities. This is one of the reasons why some people who are battling insomnia and difficulty sleeping are frequently advised to place a few drops of the oil on their pillows every night.

Aside from sleep, lavender oil can also help release body tension and emotional stress. It lowers mental distractions while improving its alertness and functions. Because of this, sniffing lavender scent just before an interview or a test can help give you a more positive result. Lavender is also helpful if you're battling with frequent migraine attacks.

For headaches, you can massage a few drops of lavender directly on your temples. You can also add a few drops of the oil to a basin of water. Dip a washcloth in the water and wring out any excess. For best effect, you can lie down for a couple of minutes and cover your forehead with the towel.

Jasmine Essential Oil

Jasmine is a potent anti-anxiety essential oil. It's been called the 'king of oils" for the great things it can do. Experts are likening its effect to Valium, a potent drug in managing anxiety disorders and symptoms of alcohol withdrawal. It specifically targets the activity of GABA, an innate brain activity inhibitor, to lower over-excitement and stress.

To experience the benefits of Jasmine oil, you can use a diffuser. It helps quickly distribute the scent. You can also add the oil in a warm bath at night to relieve tension and depression. For a quick fix, you can mix it with a carrier oil and indulge in an aromatherapy massage.

Chamomile Essential Oil

Chamomile teas are effective in calming stress and tension. When used as an essential oil, chamomile is also great in relieving anxiety and insomnia. It has a sweet and fruity scent which you can easily recognize and appreciate.

Aside from adding it to your diffuser, you can also apply chamomile essential oil directly on your feet right before you sleep. You can also create a calming salve by combining chamomile oil with coconut oil.

Essential Oils for Pain Management

One of the earliest uses of essential oils involves pain relief. Older cultures and civilizations didn't have the type of medical knowledge we have today. Instead of apparatus and bottles of medicines, they kept certain amounts of essential oils at home to remedy pain and discomfort.

Eucalyptus Essential Oil

Eucalyptus has a potent anti-inflammatory and analgesic properties. Because of this, it's widely used in managing sprain, nerve pain and muscle aches. Its most common method of application is massage. It can also be added to your warm bath for extra benefits.

Eucalyptus is also good to use in pain associated with wounds and scrapes. Aside from providing pain relief, it's also effective in keeping infections at bay due to its antiseptic properties. It also gives off a cool and refreshing feeling to help ease away the uncomfortable symptoms of arthritis.

Juniper Essential Oil

Juniper oil is one of the most popular essential oils that can help keep pain away. Specifically, it works best in managing arthritis, nerve and joint pains. It's even useful for people who are suffering from painful urination and those with hemorrhoids.

Juniper oil's mechanism of action involves an increase in blood circulation and decrease in inflammation. These two properties are essential in keeping the stubborn symptoms of arthritis at bay. By increasing blood flow, the oil is also helpful in relieving muscle fatigue and swelling.

To experience the benefits of this oil, you can apply it directly on the affected areas. You can also add it in your bath water or create a cream that has a juniper oil base. In relieving pain associated with hemorrhoids, you can add a few drops of the oil in your Hot Sitz water. You have to keep in mind, however, that the recommended maximum time for this treatment is around 20 minutes.

Sandalwood Essential Oil

Sandalwood is another great oil to use when you're in pain. It's most commonly used in relaxing muscle spasms, managing pain in sciatica and in relieving inflammation in general. It's also effective in relieving almost all types of cramps.

The oil can be applied topically on the affected area to achieve quick results. You have the option to use it as it is or to mix it with separate carrier oil. You can, however, just soak yourself in a sandalwood bath if your body is aching from overexertion or too much physical stress. This method is more commonly used by athletes after engaging in a hard day's work out or activity.

Before using the oil, make sure to test a small area on your skin for any sensitivity reaction. If you are pregnant or planning to use the oil on your younger child, then you should stick with using something else. The oil should also be avoided by people suffering from kidney disorders and other similar medical conditions.

Essentials Oils for Skin Health

Women of earlier cultures indulge their skin on essential oils and their benefits. Their skin care routine is as not as advanced and complicated as the ones we have now, yet their skin reflected health, purity and youth. Because of these, a lot of people are finding inspiration on the way they took care of their skin. Essential oils are surely penetrating today's women's beauty arsenals.

Rose Essential Oil

Rose oil is, perhaps, one of the best essential oils you can use on your skin. Because it offers a lot of benefits, it isn't surprising to find tons of skin care products infusing it as one of their main ingredients.

The oil offers a lot in terms of keeping your skin healthy. It has a supplementing effect by increasing the permeability of your skin. This means that rose oil, when applied before any product, greatly enhances the product's absorption into the skin. As a result, you get the maximum benefit of your creams and lotions.

Rose oil is also great to use if you're suffering from acne and breakouts. Because it has a strong antimicrobial property, your skin's capability to resist bacterial proliferation greatly increases. For this purpose, you may need to dab the oil twice or thrice a day on your face. For overall skin benefit, you can apply rose oil on your face and neck every morning and before you go to bed at night.

Carrot Seed Essential Oil

Carrot seed oil is slowly gaining popularity in the skin care market. It's most known for its anti-aging and potent antioxidant content. The oil promises to keep your skin young looking and wrinkle free.

Carrot seed oil can help reverse the damages done by the free radicals in your system. It also aids in better detoxification to help flush toxins off of your body. Toxin buildups are one of the most common reasons why you're experiencing frequent breakouts and acne attacks.

To keep you looking fresh, carrot seed oil helps prevent wrinkle formation. It enhances your skin's natural protection to slow down the signs of skin aging. In case you're battling with acne scars, you can also use this oil to diminish its appearance.

Geranium Essential Oil

If you're troubled with a bad case of acne, using geranium oil can be helpful. By regulating oil production, this oil can help control unwanted breakouts. It can improve the tone of your skin as well as its elasticity.

Because of these properties, geranium oil can be your skin's best friend. This oil's effect is not only limited to preventing acne formation. It's also good in repairing damages such as broken capillaries and bruises. By increasing circulation, you can expect these issues to be resolved in no time.

To reap these benefits, you can mix geranium with a carrier oil before applying it on your face. You can also create your own toner by mixing it with distilled water. If you have stubborn scars that you want out of your life, simply dab a small amount of the oil and leave it on your skin overnight.

Essential Oils for Improved Immune System

Perhaps, the best and most popular use of essential oils, next to skin care, is general health. People who detest taking chemically prepared medications opt to use essential oils in treating minor ailments and in boosting their health. If you are one of these people, then the following oils can surely set you off the right track towards a stronger immune system.

Tea Tree Essential Oil

A low immune system can't only predispose you to simple cough and cold, but it can also put you at risk for several health issues. If you're looking for a natural way of improving your body's capability to fight diseases, you can start with tea tree oil.

This oil is known for its stimulating effect on the immune system. It's able to help your body defend itself against most bacteria and viruses. It also assists in cellular repair and in cellular renewal.

To enhance your immunity using tea tree oil, you can create a spray which you can use to keep your home filled with its essence. You can also pour a few drops of the oil and massage it on the soles of your feet. You can apply the oil on its own. However, if you have sensitive skin, it's best if you can mix tea tree with another oil to dilute it. Coconut and jojoba oil are the most recommended for this purpose. This oil must never be taken internally, in any way.

Bay Laurel Essential Oil

Laurel leaf essential oil is another oil that works to supplement your immune system. People who are frequently exposed to stress and changes in environment can most benefit from using it. It has properties that can prevent flu, bacterial infections and even respiratory viruses.

Laurel oil works to prevent health issues. It's not suitable to use as a remedy for an already existent illness. If your interest is piqued by this oil, be sure to grab one that's certified therapeutic grade. It shouldn't be used by children as young as six years old and below. Pregnant women should also skip using this essential oil.

Castor Seed Essential Oil

Castor oil has a lot to offer in terms of taking care of your health. One of its most known benefits involves stimulating your immune system. By triggering your lymphatic system to dispose accumulated toxins and to synthesize more lymphocytes, castor oil can greatly improve your ability to ward off infections and diseases.

Aside from flushing toxins, this oil can also prevent and suppress any possible bacterial proliferation in your system. It also increases your body's blood circulation which, in turn, allows your body organs to function at their optimum level. Castor oil is effective not only in fighting against bacteria, it's also equally efficient in killing viruses and fungi.

The oil is best used as an oil pack. You can use either a hot water bottle or a simple cloth drenched with the essence. Most people saw and felt positive results after using the pack three to four times a week for one whole month.

To create a castor oil pack is easy. For the procedure, you need to prepare a cotton or wool flannel. Grab your castor seed essential oil, a plastic wrap and a hot water bottle. After preparing these materials, you can start applying oil on the cloth. Make sure that it's wet enough but not dripping. Apply the cloth over your target area. Use the plastic wrap to secure the cloth in place. When everything is settled, you can start applying minimum heat over it using the hot water bottle.

Essential Oils for Common Ailments

The benefits of using essential oils are limitless. Aside from helping you manage several serious health issues, they can also be applied to mild common ailments at home. Because chemically prepared medications can put you at certain health risks in the long run, it's best to stick with natural remedies in handling your health concerns. Aside from being a safer approach, using natural methods in healing can save you a lot of money too.

- **Clove Oil for Toothache**

Clove oil is one of the most common essential oils used in managing toothaches at home. For treatment, you'll need a piece of cotton, your clove oil and a carrier oil. Pour a few drops of the combined oil to the cotton and dab it on the affected tooth or the area around it. If you're going to apply it on the gum area, you may need to put minimum pressure.

- **Myrrh Oil for Mouth Sores**

Mouth sores can develop anywhere around and inside the oral area. They can be irritating, annoying and painful. For their treatment, the application of myrrh oil proves helpful. It has antibacterial, antiviral and even antifungal properties to help address the cause of your painful mouth sores.

The most common recipe in using myrrh oil for the treatment of mouth sores involves turning it as a mouthwash. There are a lot of variations in its preparations. However, whether you decide to include other ingredients or create a simple myrrh mouthwash, always make it a point to choose a quality myrrh oil.

- **Lemongrass Essential Oil for Fever and Flu**

Lemongrass oil has an antipyretic property. It can also relieve muscle pain and even headache. Due to these properties, lemongrass is considered effective in managing the signs of symptoms of flu or even a simple fever.

To use the oil, you need to mix it with a carrier oil. After creating the mixture, it's best applied on the feet or on the temples. Aside from lowering temperature, its effect is also soothing particularly to children.

- **Helichrysum Essential Oil for Bruises**

Bruising typically happens due to physical trauma. It usually results to a black and blue discoloration on the skin, indicating injury and broken blood vessels. Helichrysum oil works best in treating these bruises because of its ability to penetrate the deeper layers of the skin to its blood circulation where it helps hasten healing. This oil, aside from healing, also gives pain relief.

- **Calendula Essential Oil for Burns**

Burns are painful and can cause a lot of discomfort. They may take a while to heal and may even leave unattractive scars on your skin.

In addressing these issues, calendula oil is your most reliable remedy.

It helps speed up the healing process by triggering cellular growth and renewal. It has an anti-inflammatory property to minimize the pain. It also anti-septic in nature, meaning it can prevent bacterial growth and possible infections from happening.

Accidental burns aren't the only types of burn you can manage with this oil. It can also be used in treating sunburn, which is classified as first degree burn.

- **Cypress Essential Oil for Sore Throat**

Cypress oil is effective to use on sore throats because of its ability to reduce inflammation on the area as well as the associated irritation. At the first sign of sore throat, you can put a drop of the oil on your tongue. This is usually enough to provide relief. Another variation involves mixing Cypress oil with another oil or another natural ingredient. Most common choices include honey and olive oil.

Essential Oils for Digestive Health

While eating can be fulfilling and fun, nobody likes feeling bloated and cramped. To avoid these discomforts, there are essential oils you can quickly use either for fast relief or in preventing digestive issues. Here are your options:

Ginger Essential Oil

Ginger is a common kitchen staple. However, other than adding flavors to dishes, ginger has a lot of health benefits. Its essential oil, for example, can help improve your digestive health. It can help relieve indigestion, bloating and even an upset stomach. In case you are trying to gain weight, you can use this oil to stimulate your appetite.

Because it has a strong antiseptic property, ginger oil is also commonly used in managing diarrhea and even food poisoning. If you feel full with gas, you can rub a small amount of ginger oil on your abdomen. Before you prepare your ginger oil recipe, make sure you're not hypersensitive to ginger root.

Cumin Essential Oil

Cumin oil is one of the best oils to use when it comes to digestive health. Its scent alone creates an effective first stage of digestion by stimulating saliva production in your mouth. It also has thymol that directly affects the release of the necessary enzyme your digestive track needs to effectively break down food.

Cumin oil is also a good appetite stimulant. You can use it if you're trying to gain weight or just want to eat a bit more. Using cumin oil can help you avoid stomach pain, flatulence as well as indigestion.

Fennel Essential Oil

Fennel can help you attain normal bowel movement because of its laxative effect. It makes peristalsis more efficient which, in effect, stimulates your bowel to clear itself on a regular basis. It's also helpful in releasing excess gas accumulating in your stomach and in eliminating any possible worms or spores in your intestinal track.

Fennel oil can also enhance the protective layer of your stomach. It can assist in regulating the function and presence of the necessary digestive enzymes. Without these enzymes, your body will have a hard time breaking down food to a form it can easily absorb.

Essential Oils for Beautiful Hair

Because the hair is the crowning glory, you want it to become healthy, young and full of life. However, as stress and pollution seem inevitable, keeping your hair at its best condition possible can be a challenge. To win over this battle, here are the following essential oils for a beautiful mane.

Cedar wood Essential Oil

Poor blood circulation on the scalp is one of the reasons why hair thinning happens. To address this concern, you can mix cedar wood with coconut oil and generously apply them to your scalp. The act of massaging and cedar wood application improves blood flow to stimulate hair growth.

Aside from improving circulation, the oil also works to prevent any fungal infection from happening. The proliferation of fungus tends to deprive your hair the nutrients it needs to keep growing. As a result, you'll find your hair weak to the point that they easily fall off of your head.

You can massage a few drop of the oil on your hair to avoid experiencing the problem. It can be on dry or wet hair. For best result, you should leave the oil on your hair for a while.

Clary Sage Essential Oil

Clary Sage can help you keep your beautiful hair, particularly if you are the older age. Its work involves keeping your hormones' balance to make sure your hair stays at its best state. Women, who are going through the menopausal stage, are believed to benefit most from this oil.

This oil also prevents hair fall by increasing the tone of the hair follicles and skin in your scalp. Clary sage oil should not be used by pregnant women. Because it can increase toxicity level, people who are drinking alcohol should not use the oil successively.

Thyme Essential Oil

Thyme oil helps get rid of the bacteria and fungi that tend to cause infection in the scalp. These microorganisms tend to clog up pores and consume the nutrients that are meant your hair and scalp. When your hair becomes deprived of these nutrients, they become weak and fall off.

To get the best out of this oil, make sure to massage it well on your scalp. Aside from properly distributing the oil on the area, massage also stimulates blood circulation. These conditions are essential to encourage new hair growths.

Essential Oils for Allergies

Whether it's seasonal or triggered by environmental factors, experiencing allergies are never easy. Aside from constantly sneezing and rubbing your nose, teary eyes and itchiness can be really annoying. The following essential oils are good to use for people who frequently battles allergies.

Lemon Essential Oil

Lemon oil has both antihistamine and anti-inflammatory properties. These criteria are essential if you want to take care of allergies.

Lemon oil has a cooling and decongestant effect. It helps clear up your digestive track to remove excess mucus production. Aside from relieving congestion, the oil also improves blood circulation and greatly enhances the efficiency of your lymphatic system.

For allergies, you can create a spray using lemon oil. Use the spray on areas where allergens are very common, such as your pillows and sheets. If you have asthma, you can also benefit from using lemon oil particularly during seasons where pollen count is very high.

Basil Essential Oil

Basil oil can help flush out bacteria and toxins faster from your system. It can also take care of yeast and molds that can cause asthma attacks and irritation to your respiratory system. Basil oil also has a direct effect on your adrenal glands by stimulating the organs to respond properly during an allergic attack.

Basil oil can be used with vaporizers in managing respiratory issues. It has both expectorant and anti-pyretic effects to manage the fever, congestion and cough that usually accompany allergies.

Lavender Essential Oil

Lavender has the ability to reduce the swelling of your respiratory tract, a common symptom of an allergy attack. It's also effective in treating headaches caused by congestion and in calming your nerves during an attack. Other than its effect on your respiratory track, lavender oil is also helpful if your allergy is accompanied by red skin and rashes.

You can use lavender oil on its own or with a carrier oil. You can apply it on irritated areas or on your temple for instant relief. You should keep in mind, however, that lavender oil may be too strong for some people. If you are going to use it on its own, make sure to test it for skin tolerance and sensitivity first.

Essential Oils for Skin Cancer and Skin Health

Skin cancer is one of the most serious cases of cancer. It's aggressive but highly curable during the early stages. Essential oils are helpful in managing this form of cancer because they are effective and offers a natural approach of treatment.

Rosehip Essential Oil

Rosehip oil has the capability of protecting the skin against UV damage. It can fight free radicals and prevent them from doing harm on your skin's elastin. It has both antiseptic and anti-inflammatory effects to manage the signs and symptoms associated with skin cancer. It's also capable of increasing your melanin production.

The oil has potent components that can prevent cancer from happening in the first place. It's rich in antioxidant contents such as catechins, flavonoids and polyphenols. It also has a good anti-aging effect by stimulating collagen formation. Collagen not only helps counter fine lines and wrinkles, but it's also helpful in filling up indented scars.

Lemon Essential Oil

Lemon oil is, perhaps, one of the most researched and proven oil that can help remedy cancer. Its effect is not only limited to skin cancer but it can help even in managing cancer of the cervix.

Lemon oil has been established to block the spread of cancer cells. It's also noted for stopping free radicals from causing damage to your body's healthy cells. Other anti-cancer mechanisms of lemon oil include cellular apoptosis and inhibition of cell cycle.

You can use lemon oil solely in battling with cancer cells. However, there are other cells that can enhance its effect. Some of these oil include lemongrass and clove lead. These oils are also beneficial for cancer patients who are suffering from nausea and vomiting.

A recent study suggests that the scent of lemon oil alone can also help win over cancer. The smell of lemon is associated with that citronella terpenes can help cancer cell metastases. Receptors for these terpenes are widely distributed over the body.

Frankincense Essential Oil

Aside from its ability to enhance your immune system, frankincense oil can also help you fight cancer. It's most notable mechanisms against malignancy involve increasing lymphocytes and reducing inflammation.

The problem, however, with using Frankincense is its ability to aggravate bleeding tendencies. If you are taking any blood thinners or suffering from bleeding disorders, then it's best if you can take the use of Frankincense off of your treatment

Undiluted Frankincense, when applied directly, can help heal skin cancer spots. It usually needs 2 to 3 drops for higher efficacy.

Essential Oils for Pets

Humans aren't the only ones who can benefit from essential oils. Research suggests that there are also tons of benefits of these wonder oils to your most beloved animal friends. Here are some of them:

Cats

Cats often display sensitivity issues when it comes to being exposed to essential oils. Aside from their highly sensitive nose, their skin is also prone to overexposure because of its thinness. Even a small amount of concentrated essential oil can easily disturb their systems.

Oregano Essential Oil

A lot of cat owners use oregano oil in treating digestive problems. It is also often used topically to treat a number of skin conditions. Although there are reports that applying oregano oil works, there are still a lot of concerns about its use.

For one, oregano oil can be stingy when applied on the skin. There's also the risk of causing tongue burns in case your cat does happen to lick the oil off of his skin. There are even cats who displayed lack of appetite for several days after being exposed to the oil.

Although oregano oil can be effective and is all natural, if you have other treatment options, you should stick with the safer alternative.

Lavender Essential Oil

The application of lavender oil is most common among stressed and anxious cats. It's best applied when your pet will be separated from you for a while or when he's faced with a stressful situation. Pet owners usually dispense a small amount of the oil behind their cats' ears and paw pads. The remaining oil on their hands is rubbed along their spine.

Lavender oil is also good to use to relieve dry and itchy skin. It can also be used in managing irritated and painful skin. If your cat has minor wounds, applying this oil can help in regeneration and fast healing.

Spearmint Essential Oil

Spearmint oil is widely used in treating digestive issues among cats. Aside from this purpose, the oil is also helpful in regulating digestion, reducing colic and in losing weight.

Dogs

Chamomile Essential Oil

Chamomile oil is helpful in relieving anxiety in dogs. It's gentle and has an analgesic effect on animals. If your dog is suffering from spasms and cramps, using chamomile can really help. Chamomile oil also has anti-parasitic and anti-inflammatory effects. With caution, it can be taken internally or applied topically.

Eucalyptus Essential Oil

Instead of using chemical based flea treatment, you can go for a more natural approach by using eucalyptus oil instead. It's best used when mixed with your dog's existing shampoo. After lathering the eucalyptus shampoo on your dog, let it sit for around two minutes. This is done to help the essential oil work its way to your dog's skin. After rinsing, you may want to repeat the process for best result.

Frankincense Essential Oil

This oil is commonly used in dogs with cancer. It helps enhance canine immune system and to reduce the size of cancer cells. Using this, however, requires extra caution. Frankincense is known as a potent cerebral vasodilator. One of its effect include high blood pressure.

Helichrysum Essential Oil

Most commonly used as a first aid in emergencies, helichrysum oil is effective in controlling bleeding. It's also useful in nerve repair and in assisting recovery from cardiac diseases.

Typically, the way aromatherapy and essential oils affect humans is the same for dogs. If you see them lively and in a good mood, then the oils could be doing them right. However, if you find your dog irritable, drooling or shying away from the scent, then it means they're reacting negatively to it.

It can also help if you can give your pets a rest period in between use of essential oils. This rest period is necessary in keeping toxicity and sensitivity issues away. This gap may take one or two weeks of not using essential oil.

However, for certain health issues, such as cancer, the use of essential oil must be carried on for a longer period of time. In these instances, treatment must be left on the hands of trained and skilled professionals. They are the best people who can render the best effects of essential oil without putting your pets' lives at risk.

Essential Oils for Massage

Essential oils are widely used in aromatherapy massages. Aside from the physical benefits, these oils can do wonders for your mental and emotional health. Here are some of the best essential oils you can use:

Mandarin Essential Oil

Mandarin oil, when used in aromatherapy massage, can relax your muscles because of its antispasmodic effects. It helps release you muscle tension while providing you with an instant mood enhancer. Other than its direct effect on your muscles, it has a sedative effect too. It can help you feel calmer and sleep better.

The oil can also improve blood circulation which is why it's frequently the oil of choice among people with painful joints and arthritis. When massaged on your abdominal area, lemon oil can help relieve gastritis and other stomach discomfort.

Mandarin oil may cause photosensitivity reactions. After applying the oil, make sure to avoid exposing yourself to direct sunlight for a couple of hours to avoid redness and possible blister formations.

Marjoram Essential Oil

Marjoram oil is mostly used to soothe muscle right after an intense workout or physical activity. It relaxes tense muscles and supports the functions of the cardiovascular system. While it smells spice and woody, marjoram oil has a calming effect.

Preparing marjoram oil needs extra caution particularly in people with sensitive skin. Most of the time, it's prepared on a 50:50 method with one part essential oil and another part from a carrier or vegetable oil. You can massage the mixture directly on target areas to get instant relief.

Eucalyptus Essential Oil

Eucalyptus, when used in aromatherapy massage, can help relieve respiratory issues, joint problems and muscle pain. It's usually massaged in a circular motion to obtain the best effect.

In people with asthma, two drops of this oil is usually massaged on the chest area to help relieve congestion and to dilate the bronchial tubes. Because of this dilation, a larger amount of oxygen is able to reach the lungs.

Essential Oils for Kids

While essential oils are beneficial, not all are safe enough to be applied or used on your child's sensitive skin. Before addressing what type of oil you can or can't use, you might want to take a look at this guideline first:

- Essential oils should not be applied to your child if he is less than three months. At this age, his skin is still fragile and highly permeable to what you apply on it.

- If your child is older than three months and essential oils are necessary, keep in mind to introduce one oil at a time. This is done to help determine any sensitivity reaction your kid has. One oil per day is usually enough to allow reactions to surface, if there are any.

- Do not use an undiluted essential oil on kids. As a matter of fact, all oils should be diluted if they are going to be used among the young ones. You can dilute it in honey or in vegetable.

- Avoid applying the oil directly or anywhere near your kid's nose. The best places to start essential oil application are the feet, hands and chest.

- Clove essential oil may be too strong for the kids and must be avoided until they are 2 years old and above.

- Peppermint and eucalyptus are also not recommended to use either topically or by inhalation to children under 6 years old. The oil's menthol content may be too much to cause slowed respiration or bradypnea in children.

- Inhalation might be the best way to use essential oils in children.

- Wintergreen essential oil is not recommended to use on children because of its methylsalicylate content.

After reading these guidelines, here's the list of essential oils you can use on your child and at what age you can safely introduce them.

- For babies who are only 3 months of age, Chamomile, Lavender and Dill are safe options.

- If your child is 6 months or older, Lemon and Cinnamon bark are safe to use by diffusion.

- For children 6 months older, topical application of Cedar wood, Geranium, and Neroli essential oil are safe.

- Children who've reached 2 years of age can use Juniper, Basil and Myrrh either by diffusion or topical application.

As kids are innately active, you should also keep in mind sun exposure. There are actually a lot of essential oils that cause photosensitivity and sensitivity reactions. Bergamot, Grapefruit and Orange essential oils are some of them.

Chapter 4

Best Ways to Use Essential Oils

Picking the right essential oil can be both tricky and fun. However, finding out how you should use your essential oil can be challenging. To give you a clearer idea of your options, this section will help you learn the best ways you can use your favorite essential oil.

Massage

Massage is one of the most common and effective ways you can introduce an essential oil to your system. Aside from the actual benefits of the oil, you also get an improved blood circulation. Massage triggers and stimulates your skin, nerves and muscles. Depending on your need, you can use one or more essential oils. You may also need to dilute based on your skin's sensitivity and reaction.

Compress

The use of compress is highly effective when it comes to essential oil use. They are often used for first aid in minor emergencies such as sprains, bruises and localized swelling. Depending on the case, you may need to choose between a hot and a cold essential oil compress. As a rule of thumb, warm compresses are used when dealing with abscesses and menstrual cramps. For cold compresses, sprains are the most common type of emergency they're applied.

Inhalation

For congestion and difficulty breathing, inhalation can be your best method particularly during the cold and winter season. For this method, you only need a large bowl, hot water, a towel and your essential oil. Pour a few drops of your essential oil to the water filled bowl. Eucalyptus and Peppermint oils are the most common essential oils to be used for the approach. To catch the steam and the essence of the oil, you need to pull the towel over your head and lean over the bowl. Practice caution when using this technique as burns is relatively common.

Gargle

Essential oils can also be used as gargles particularly if you're suffering from swollen gums and toothaches. Tea tree oil is one of the most common oils used for this method. It's typically mixed with water and honey for increased efficacy. To get the most out of it, make sure to repeat this process once every four hours.

Bath

To combat stress, indulging in an essential oil bath once in a while could help. As the benefits of the oils penetrate your skin, you can also enjoy the aroma in your bath. The best oil for this method depends on what purpose you want the bath to serve. To wake you up, Citrus oil bath could help. However, if you're aiming to get a better sleep at night, Chamomile or Lavender oil work best. Keep in mind that the maximum recommended drops for bath is around 6 to 8. Anything more than that can be drying for the skin.

Vapor

To spread the scent and benefits of your essential oil, you can use a vaporizer or a burner. You can choose to go natural or buy an electric one. The use of vapor is particularly useful among sick individuals who are at risk for airborne pathogens while recovering.

In choosing the best vaporizer, there are criteria you can use to pick out the best one for your home. Aside from determining a vaporizer's capacity, you also need to have a good idea on how far its range is. You want to find a device that can sufficiently cover your room. There are also diffusers today that come with good lightings to greatly enhance the therapeutic effect of the oils.

Chapter 5

How to Take Care of Your Essential Oils

There's more to essential oils than their purpose. As a matter of fact, the way they were created, stored and kept plays a crucial role on how good their effects can be. For your essential oils to stay in their best state here are a few things to remember.

Storage

- Essential oils must be kept in a dry and cool place.

- Some oils are sensitive to light. Be careful where you place them.

- You can store your oils inside your refrigerator or in places where changes in temperature isn't likely to happen.

- For containers, it's best to keep them in amber or cobalt blue bottles. Amber bottles are more affordable than the blue ones.

- Avoid including a rubber dropper in your bottle. Always choose a screw cap to keep your oils secure and fresh.

Disposal

- Essential oils are volatile. Avoid disposing them in flames.

- You also should readily pour all your oils down your drain, particularly if there's a chance for the oils to get in contact with your water supply.

- One of the most recommended ways of disposing essential oils is by pouring the oil in an inert object and then sealing both off in a special container.

- Another option involves allowing the essential oil to evaporate on baking soda.

If you still have a good amount of essential oil left, you have the option to reuse it for a different purpose. You can use a small amount to freshen up your drain. While pouring a large quantity of oil down your drain is not recommended, a small amount of the same oil isn't bad either. You can compare this amount to the content most soap and skin products have that gets carried down the drain when you wash yourself or take a shower.

You can also use the remaining essential oil on your seasonal clothing. This helps keep bad odor away until you're ready to use the clothes again. Storage boxes and cabinets can also benefit from the oil. You can also use the same oil to freshen up your trash bin. To help improve the smell of your laundry, you can add it to your homemade fabric softener.

Reusing Old Essential Oil Bottles

There are a lot of ways you can recycle your old essential oil bottles. In case you're planning on reusing it for your next batch of essential oil, then you need to make sure there are no residues of its previous contents. Here's how you can thoroughly clean your bottles:

1. Take out the labels off of the bottle. Try to peel off as much as you can.

2. Disassemble the bottles and their caps. Soak everything in warm water for a couple of minutes.

3. To remove the sticky labels entirely, you can add a few drops of lemon oil to the water.

4. After the labels have been thoroughly remove, soak them again in a different bowl of water with a good household cleaner.

5. Rinse the bottles and caps and allow them to dry in air.

There are exciting and creative ways for you to reuse your old bottles. It may not necessarily be about using them for essential oils. For other ideas, here's a short list you can use:

- Old bottles can be used as gift containers. You can use it to share your essential oils or other DIY concoctions with friends.

- You can also use it as storage in case you're travelling. It's never fun to carry big bags and luggage just to accommodate your whole collection of essential oils while travelling across the country.

- These small containers can also be used in storing your homemade bath salts.

Conclusion

Essential oils can do a lot of things for you and your health. Although they are an age-old approach to taking care of your body, they are still effective and generally a lot safer than what we have today. They may require a bit of research, understanding and interest before you can fully reap their benefits. As one essential oil is different from another, you want to find the best one that can give you exactly what you need and what you want.

There are no short cuts to getting healthier and more beautiful. There aren't any overnight miracles, too. However, with the right essential oil and the right technique, you are surely set to be on your best state possible.